50 Best Body Scrub Recipes

By Emma Curtis

Visit: EmmasTake.WordPress.com

About Emma

Emma Curtis is an animal lover, green living guru, and user of chemical-free beauty products. With her clean eating plans, healthy homemade recipes, and fantastic workout routines, you'll be on your way to a healthier, happier, and greener life in no time at all!

Please & Thank You

Before we begin, I'd love to take this opportunity to thank you for purchasing this book and also ask that you please share it with your friends. If you enjoy it, taking a moment to leave a review would brighten my day!

As always, my mission is to help others live happier, healthier lives. Seeing my readers' creations and pretty faces never fails to bring instant joy to my heart, so if you have anything to add or simply want to post a picture or share a quote, please feel free to do so at my blog: EmmasTake.WordPress.com.

Let's get started!

Emma

Table of Contents

What & Why

The body scrubs in this book will be made from sugar, salt, or oatmeal. All body scrubs are perfect for rejuvenating your skin and treating yourself to a wonderful at-home spa day!

Whether you have only heard about body scrubs from a friend or have had the pleasure of trying one yourself, these recipes are sure to delight you!

Body scrubs can be used regularly, especially for those suffering from dry skin. To use a body scrub, simply apply it in a circular motion, starting at your ankles and working all the way up. Focus some extra attention on your dry skin patches, such as your elbows and hands.

The wonderful thing about body scrubs is that you can make them in practically any scent! This book is organized into multiple categories, such as fresh and sweet, autumn, chocolate, and holiday scents so you can easily locate whatever you desire.

Here are some tips before you begin…

1. Mason jars are the best place to store your body scrubs. Clean out jam jars well before use to ensure the scents don't mix!

2. It can get slippery in the tub, so be careful and invest in a non-slip mat.

3. Some scrubs can be formed into solid bars, while others will be more liquid and need to be applied with a bath cloth or scrubby. Use both and see which one you prefer!

4. There are so many different scents and recipes, and each one has a dozen variations! Experiment and have fun with it!

5. Exact measurements aren't a necessity with these recipes, so don't worry if you're a bit off.

6. Prepare a scrub, decorate a jar, and it will make the perfect gift for just about anybody you know who bathes (which I hope is everybody!).

Fresh & Sweet Scents

These recipes feature sweet and fresh fragrances, such as grapefruit and orange vanilla. Scents like these are perfect for warmer months, but you can of course use them whenever you're wanting a tropical-themed spa shower!

1: Whipped Grapefruit Mint Sugar Scrub

Ingredients:

- ½ cup Coconut Oil
- ½ cup White Sugar
- Zest of 1 Grapefruit
- 1 T. Grapefruit Juice
- 10 drops Peppermint Oil
- 25 drops Grapefruit Oil
- ¼ t. Beet Juice (optional, for color only)

Directions:

1. Make sure your coconut oil is firm. Place it in a bowl with the white sugar and mix. Continue until it has reached the consistency of a thick paste.
2. Add in the grapefruit juice and zest, along with the peppermint and grapefruit oil. If desired, add beat juice as well.
3. Blend on medium until your mixture is blended and fluffy.
4. Use as desired and store in an air-tight glass dry inside refrigerator.

2: Navel Orange Vanilla Sugar Scrub

Ingredients:

- ¼ cup virgin coconut oil
- ¼ cup raw sugar
- 1 tablespoon Paramount Citrus navel orange zest
- ½ of a vanilla bean

Directions:

1. In a medium bowl, add the coconut oil, raw sugar, and orange zest.
2. Use a knife to slit the center of the vanilla bean. Using the tip of the knife, scrape out the paste and put it into the bowl.
3. Mix it all together until everything is combined nicely. Make sure the vanilla is distributed evenly in the scrub.
4. Store in a sealed container, like an eight-ounce canning jar.

I typically use a teaspoon and spread it over my hands or feet, then rinse with warm water and pat dry with a soft towel.

3: Paradise Mango Scrub

Ingredients:

- 1/2 cup raw sugar
- 2 tablespoons coconut oil (if solid, heat in microwave)
- 1/4 cup chopped raw mango
- 3-4 drops of orange essential oil

Directions:

1. Mash all the ingredients together, add more sugar and oil until the consistency is thick.
2. Apply starting at your feet in a circular motion. Use your hands or a scrubby or cloth.

This is one of my favorite summer scents!

4: Sweet Grape Body Scrub

Ingredients:

- 3 cups sugar
- 1-2 teaspoons grape drink mix
- 2 ½ cups of coconut oil

Directions:

1. Stir together the sugar with 1 teaspoon of drink mix to start, adding more as needed.
2. Once combined, add in the oil and mix again.

Make sure to store this in an airtight container. This recipes makes a good amount, so there's plenty to share! It's great for a girls' night. I wasn't so sure about grape when I first tried it, but it's now one of my top fruit-scented recipes.

5: Green Tea Body Scrub

Ingredients:

- 1 cup granulated white sugar
- ½ cup coconut oil
- 1 Tablespoon green tea
- 1 teaspoon green tea powder

Directions:

1. Gather all of your ingredients and measure accordingly.
2. Combine them all in a bowl and mix thoroughly.
3. Be sure to use an airtight container to store this between uses!

Green tea is always refreshing, whether you're drinking it or applying it! It also has many health benefits, like:

- Better brain function
- Fat loss!
- Lowered risk of cancer
- It may reduce your risk of Alzheimer's, Parkinson's disease, type II diabetes, and even cardiovascular disease!

6: Coconut Milk Sugar Scrub

Ingredients:

- 1/2 cup coconut milk
- 1/2 cup turbinado sugar
- 1 tablespoon of coconut oil

Directions:

1. Mix all together! If your coconut oil is solid, heat in the microwave for a few seconds.
2. Store (as always) in an airtight container (if there's any left!).

Random quote about true beauty...

"For beautiful eyes, look for the good in others; for beautiful lips, speak only words of kindness; and for poise, walk with the knowledge that you are never alone."

~Audrey Hepburn

7: Coconut Lime Sugar Scrub

Ingredients:

- 1 cup coconut oil
- 1.5 cup sugar
- zest from one lime
- lime essential oil

Directions:

1. Combine the oil, lime zest, and sugar together.
2. Start with seven drops of the lime oil, adding more a drop at a time until you're happy with the strength of the scent.
3. Put it in a glass jar!

Benefits of Coconut Oil...

Coconut oil not only smells amazing, it also has some amazing health benefits, just like green tea! Here are just a few reasons to use it more...

1. For reasons that are known, populations who enjoy coconut on a regular basis are among the healthiest nations on the

planet! For instance, the Tokelauans (in the South Pacific) eat tons of coconut. Their health is generally excellent and there are no known cases of heart disease!

2. This is likely because coconut oil increases the amount of energy your body burns, resulting in less fat!

3. The Lauric Acid in coconut oil kills bacteria, viruses, and fungi!

4. Coconut oil kills your hunger, so it's a great thing to have around if you get the munchies often...

5. The fatty acids present in coconut oil are converted into Ketones by your body, which reduce the chance of a seizure!

8: Snow Cone Sugar Scrub

Ingredients:

- 3 tablespoons coconut oil
- 2 teaspoons almond oil
- 1/3 cup granulated sugar

Directions:

This recipe is beautiful when food coloring is added, making for a true snow cone appearance. Follow these directions for each color:

1. Mix all ingredients listed above for each color.
2. Add a couple drops of flavored oil of your choice for the scent.
3. Mix in a couple drops of food coloring and apply!

Hint...

With recipes featuring coconut (there are so many!) it might harden while being stored, but will typically soften again in the temperature of your hands or warm water, so don't worry!

9: Coconut Birthday Cake Sugar Scrub

Ingredients:

- ¼ cup turbinado sugar
- ¼ cup dark brown sugar
- ¼ cup sugar
- ¼ cup coconut butter
- 1 teaspoon vanilla extract
- ¼ teaspoon almond extract

Directions:

1. Combine all sugars in a bowl and stir.
2. Add coconut butter along with the extracts.
3. Use as you desire!

10: Lemon Poppy seed Scrub

Ingredients:

- 1 cup caster sugar
- 3 table spoons of almond or coconut oil
- 8 drops of lemon essential oil
- 1 table spoon of poppy seeds
- zest of one lemon

Directions:

1. Put the sugar, poppy seeds, and lemon zest into a bowl and mix until it's evenly combined.
2. Add the almond and lemon oils, mixing again. Now you should have a mixture about the consistency of moist sand.
3. Cover with lid and enjoy!

11: Himalayan Pink Salt Scrub

Ingredients:

- 8 ounces pink Himalayan sea salt
- 2 ounces coconut oil
- 1 ounce sweet almond oil
- 10 drops rose geranium essential oil
- 5 drops citrus essential oil
- 5 drops ylang ylang essential oil

Directions:

1. Mix all the ingredients together in a jar!
2. Apply!

This would make a wonderful gift, as all of these scrubs would. If you plan on giving it away, some rose petals on top would make it that much cuter!

12: Citrus Salt Body Scrub

Ingredients:

- 1/2 cup sea salt
- 1/2 cup jojoba, almond, or olive oil
- 1 teaspoon orange or grapefruit zest

Directions:

1. Combine the sea salt and oil together.
2. Add in the zest and make sure everything is saturated.
3. Store in a jar, use all over your body and towel dry afterwards.

13: Almond and Floral Body Scrub

Ingredients:

- 1 cup sea salt (or epsom salt)
- 1/2 cup a sweet almond oil
- 6 drops to 1/4 teaspoon of floral oil (like geranium oil)
- 1/4 cup lavender buds
- fresh flower petals (optional)

Directions:

1. Mix everything together.
2. Store in jar!

These recipes will last a little while in the fridge, but being that most of them use fresh ingredients, it's a good idea to use them within a week of preparation (which shouldn't be a problem, right?!).

14: Rose Body Scrub

Ingredients:

- Fine sea salt
- Coarse sea salt (himalayan salt)
- Rose essential oil
- Jojoba Oil

Directions:

1. Mix the salts together first.
2. Add the jojoba oil (or any other unscented oil).
3. Add the rose oil as desired.

You want your bath scrub to be in-between, not too wet and not too dry.

15: Pina Colada Coconut & Lemon scrub

Ingredients:

- 1 cup Dessicated Coconut
- 1 cup Epsom Salts
- 2 tablespoons of Coconut Oil (available at Heath Food Shops)
- 4 drops Vitamin E Oil (optional)
- 1 Lemon (peel finely grated)

Directions:

1. Combine the dry ingredients together in a bowl.
2. Add in the coconut oil until you reach the desired consistency.
3. Store in a container!

You always want to make sure your skin is wet before exfoliating with a body scrub. These are perfect to use after (or while) soaking in the tub or taking a nice shower.

16: Ginger Detox Body Scrub

Ingredients:

- 1 tablespoon fresh ginger
- ½ cup of Epsom salt
- 1 tablespoon lemon juice

Directions:

1. Combine the roughly chopped ginger and salt in a food processer. Pulse until the ginger is finely chopped and combined well.
2. Put into a small bowl and add the lemon juice.
3. Store in a jar.

Aren't these recipes incredibly simple? Body scrubs are some of the easiest of all beauty recipes, and they do wonders for your skin and soul.

17; Mint Lime Salt Scrub

Ingredients:

- Coconut oil
- Epsom salt
- Lime extract
- Peppermint extract

Directions:

1. The ratio we'll use for this recipe is approximately two parts oil for every one part of salt. But, as I said at the start, none of these measurements have to be perfect!
2. Melt the coconut oil.
3. Mix with salt.
4. Stir in extracts and enjoy!

18: Sea Shower Scrub

Ingredients:

- 3 tablespoons fine sea salt
- 1 tablespoon juice of a lemon
- 1 tablespoon orange blossom water (or another blossom, like rose water)
- 1 tablespoon coconut oil

Directions:

1. Add the coconut oil and salt, stirring very well.
2. Add the lemon or lime juice, mixing again.
3. Add in the blossom water until it looks really moist!
4. If you want, add some blue food coloring for a fun color!

Why salt scrubs?

You know another great think about using salt-based body scrubs? Salt dissolves in water, which means no clogged drains!

19: Geranium Pink Sea Salt Body Scrub

Ingredients:

- 1 cup Pink Himalayan Salt (Extra-Fine Grain)
- 1/2 cup Organic Coconut Oil
- 10-20 drops Geranium Essential Oil

Directions:

1. Combine the sea salt and coconut oil in a bowl.
2. Add in the oil.
3. Spoon into a jar and store!

20: Ultimate Skin Scrub (With Frankincense)

Ingredients:

- 1 cup organic brown sugar
- 2 tablespoons fine dead sea salt
- 2 tablespoons fine himalayan salt
- 2 tablespoons almond oil
- 2 tablespoons avocado oil
- 2 tablespoons grapeseed oil
- 2 tablespoon jojoba oil
- 2 tablespoons raw honey
- 1 teaspoon vitamin e oil
- 15 drops frankincense essential oil
- 8 drops lavender essential oil
- 8 drops ylang ylang essential oil

Directions:

1. Start by mixing the sugar and salts.
2. Pour in the liquids, putting the oils on top.
3. To use, add a few drops of water and apply.

21: Oatmeal Honey Scrub

Ingredients:

- 2 parts oatmeal (finely ground in a blender or food processor)
- 1 part honey
- 1 part sweet almond oil (or coconut or olive oil)

Directions:

1. Mix it all up!
2. You want the consistency of a thick, sticky mixture.

This is perfect as a face scrub after a long day!

22: Coconut Oatmeal Scrub

Ingredients:

- 1 1/2 cup oatmeal
- 1/2 cup organic coconut oil
- 1 teaspoon vanilla extract
- 1 teaspoon honey
- 1 teaspoon brown sugar

Directions:

1. Ground up the oatmeal in your food processor, then place into a bowl.
2. Add the brown sugar.
3. Pour in the coconut oil, honey, and vanilla and mix!

23: Rose + Chamomile Scrub

Ingredients:

- 1 tablespoon dried roses
- 1 tablespoon dried chamomile
- 1 tablespoon oats
- 2 tablespoons honey
- 1/4 cup of mild oil (almond, olive, jojoba, sesame)

Directions:

1. In a coffee grinder, combine the oatmeal and dried flowers.
2. Transfer to your container and add the honey and oil.

This one, like many, is mild enough to use all over multiple times a week! When sealed in an airtight container, because of the dry, natural ingredients, this one can last practically forever as long as no water gets into the jar, but I think you'll use it long before then!

24: Oatmeal Almond Body Scrub

Ingredients:

- 2/3 cup almonds {whole, slivers, slices, whatever you have}
- 2/3 cup oatmeal
- 1/2 cup brown sugar
- 1/4 cup olive oil
- 1/4 cup coconut oil
- 2 tablespoon honey
- 1 teaspoon vanilla

Directions:

1. In a coffee grinder or food processor, grind the oatmeal and almonds.
2. Mix the remaining ingredients in a bowl.
3. Store in a tight-fitting jar.

25: Oatmeal & Honey Sugar Scrub

Ingredients:

- ½ cup oats
- ¼ cup baby oil
- 1 ¼ cup sugar
- ¼ honey

Directions:

1. Combine!
2. Store in a jar and enjoy as you wish.

26: Oatmeal Body Scrub

Ingredients:

- 1 cup coconut oil
- ½ cup brown sugar
- ½ cup finely ground oatmeal
- 1-2 tablespoons olive oil

Directions:

1. Using your coffee grinder, blender, or food processer, pulse the oats until they're powdered (you'll still have a few small pieces).
2. Combine the oils, sugar, and oats in a bowl.
3. Pour the scrub into jars and enjoy!

27: Oatmeal Cookie Scrub

Ingredients:

- ¾ cup oatmeal, ground finely
- 2 tablespoons brown sugar
- 2 tablespoons white sugar
- 1 tablespoon baking soda
- 7 tablespoons carrier oil (coconut, sweet almond, sunflower)

Directions:

1. Grind the oatmeal until you have a powder consistency
2. Combine and mix all the dry ingredients in a bowl.
3. Add in your carrier oil of choice, then store in an airtight container!

28: Pineapple Sugar Body Scrub

Ingredients:

- 1 1/2 cup cane sugar- glycolic acid
- ½ cup walnut or coconut oil
- ¼ – ½ pineapple (1/2 cup puree)

Directions:

1. Puree your pineapple until nice and smooth.
2. Add the cane sugar and oil.
3. Apply as desired and rinse with warm water.

29: Mango Body Scrub for Sensitive Skin

Ingredients:

- 1 mango
- 2 tablespoons oats
- 1 teaspoon honey

Directions:

1. Cut the mango into chunks, then blend until smooth.
2. Mix the oats and honey in, combining well.
3. Apply as desired!

30: Papaya Sea Salt Body Scrub

Ingredients:

- ½ cup sea salt
- 1 papaya
- 2 tablespoons olive oil

Directions:

1. Cut up and blend the papaya until smooth.
2. Mix in the sea salt to make a grainy scrub.
3. If you battle oily skin, omit the olive oil!

Chocolaty Scrubs

These are perfect for the chocolate lovers among us! Here are a few of my favorite chocolate-scented scrub recipes.

31: Mint Chocolate Sugar Scrub

Ingredients:

- ½ cup brown sugar
- ½ cup white sugar
- ⅓ cup almond oil
- 2 tablespoons unsweetened cocoa powder
- 10 drops peppermint pure essential oil

Directions:

1. Add the sugars, oils, and cocoa in a large bowl, mixing well.
2. Store and use as desired!

32: Chocolate Coconut Sugar Scrub

Ingredients:

- 1 cup loosely packed brown sugar
- 1/2 cup coconut oil (in solid form)
- 1/3 cup almond oil
- 2 tablespoons unsweetened cocoa powder
- a few drops of coconut extract or essential oil

Directions:

1. Add all the ingredients and mix until they're nicely combined.
2. Store in a jar!

You can store this one at room temperature, as long as you use it all up by within a week or two. I like to sprinkle some chocolate chips on top for décor when giving as a gift.

33: Cocoa Body Scrub

Ingredients:

- ½ cup brown sugar
- 3 tablespoons cocoa powder
- ⅛ cup melted cocoa butter
- ¼ cup sweet almond oil
- Sweet orange oil essential oil (or raspberry extract or cinnamon)

Directions:

1. Melt the cocoa butter.
2. Add the powder, sugar, and oils.
3. Mix well and store!

I use a half-pint mason jar for this one, but it never lasts too long!

34: Chocolate and Coffee Sugar Scrub

Ingredients:

- 1 cup of raw sugar
- 1/2 cup of coconut oil
- 2-3 tablespoons cocoa
- 2 tablespoons ground coffee

Directions:

1. Mix all together.
2. Store in fridge.

35: Chocolate Body Scrub

Ingredients:

- 1 cup sugar
- 2 tablespoons unscented liquid soap
- 3 tablespoons cocoa powder
- 1 teaspoon vanilla extract
- olive oil

Directions:

1. Combine sugar, soap, cocoa, and vanilla.
2. Add olive oil until you reach a paste-like consistency.

Autumn & Holiday Scents

Like most everyone, the winter holidays are my favorite! Everything just seems more cheery with decorations everywhere, lights shining at night, and people thinking more about others. Here are my top holiday-themed scrubs!

36: Cinnamon Scrub

Ingredients:

- Oatmeal (or Flour if you don't have oatmeal)
- Cinnamon powder
- Warm water

Directions:

1. Put 1 teaspoon of oatmeal or flour into a bowl.
2. Add 1 teaspoon of cinnamon.
3. Add warm water until it's thick, not runny!

Here's a hint, if you over-do the water, add more flour, not cinnamon! If you're just trying this, start with half a teaspoon of cinnamon.

37: Apple Cinnamon Body Scrub

Ingredients:

- 1/4 cup brown sugar
- 1/4 cup granulated sugar
- 2 tablespoons coconut oil melted
- 1 tablespoon unsweetened applesauce
- 1/2 teaspoon cinnamon

Directions:

1. Add all ingredients and stir!
2. Store and use as desired.

38: Peppermint Scrub

Ingredients:

- 1/4 Cup of Salt
- 10 Drops Peppermint Essential Oil
- 3 Fresh Mint Leaves
- 2 Tablespoons of Jojoba Oil

Directions:

1. Chop up the mint leaves.
2. Add salt and oils.
3. Scrub! This is perfect for your feet.

39: Pumpkin Spice Sugar Scrub

Ingredients:

- 1¼ cup brown sugar
- 1 tablespoon pumpkin pie spice
- ¼ cup light olive oil (not extra virgin)
- ½ teaspoon vanilla extract

Directions:

1. Whisk together the brown sugar and pumpkin pie spice.
2. Add the oil and vanilla.

This one will keep for up to a few months at room temperature.

40: Vanilla Pumpkin Spice Sugar Scrub

Ingredients:

- 1 cup of granulated sugar
- 1/4 cup of coconut oil
- 2 teaspoon of pumpkin pie spice
- 2 teaspoons vanilla extract

Directions:

1. Just mix, and…
2. Store!

41: Gingerbread Sugar Scrub

Ingredients:

- 1 cup sugar
- 1 cup brown sugar
- 1/2 cup coconut oil (or other carrier oil)
- 1/4 cup almond oil
- 1/2 teaspoon vanilla extract
- 1/2 teaspoon cinnamon
- 1/2 teaspoon all spice
- 1/2 teaspoon ginger
- 1/2 teaspoon nutmeg

Directions:

1. Combine everything but the oils.
2. Gradually add the oils.
3. Scoop into a jar and enjoy!

42: Ginger and Coconut Oil Sugar Body Scrub

Ingredients:

- 1/4 cup coconut oil
- 1 tablespoon ginger, coarsely chopped
- 1/4 cup cold-pressed oil
- 3/4 cup granulated or turbinado sugar
- 1/4 cup kosher salt
- 1-4 drops essential oil

Directions:

1. Start by heating the coconut oil and ginger pieces on low. Heat for about five to ten minutes until the scent and juice of the ginger has mixed with the oil, then press through a coffee filter.
2. While the oil is still a little warm, add the cold-pressed oil of your choice (like tea seed, jojoba, sunflower, or almond oil)
3. Let cool to room temperature, then add sugar, salt, and essential oil (I used lemongrass).

43: Ginger Lime Coconut Body Scrub

Ingredients:

- 1/2 cup sugar
- 1/2 cup sea salt
- 1/3 cup coconut oil, melted
- 4 tablespoon olive oil
- 5 drops ginger essential oil
- 10 drops lime essential oil
- Zest from one lime (optional)

Directions:

1. Combine the sugar and salt in a small bowl.
2. Add coconut and olive oil.
3. Add remaining oils and mix well.
4. Store in container.

44: Vanilla Bean and Fresh Mint

Ingredients:

- 2 cups of coarse salt or sugar
- 1/2 cup olive oil
- 1 vanilla bean
- Large handful of fresh mint

Directions:

1. Combine the sugar or salt with the olive oil.
2. Slit the vanilla bean down the center and scrape into bowl.
3. Chop your mint leaves and put into a separate bowl.
4. Muddle the mint, then add to mixture and combine.
5. Use as desired!

More Herb Recipes

These last few recipes are my favorites when it comes to body scrubs using herbal scents…

45: Rosemary & Lemon Salt Scrub

Ingredients:

- 1 1/2 cups salt
- 4 tablespoons of olive oil
- Juice of 1-2 lemons
- Zest of one lemon
- 2 sprigs of rosemary

Directions:

1. Mix the zest of one lemon with the juice of two others.
2. Add the olive oil.
3. Let it sit while you chop your rosemary.
4. Combine it all and store in glass jar!

46: Mint & Rosemary Body Scrub

Ingredients:

- 1 cup Epsom salts
- 1/4 cup fresh rosemary
- 1 cup pure grape seed oil
- 20-30 drops pure rosemary essential oil
- 20 drops pure peppermint essential oil

Directions:

1. Mix all together, making sure you chop the rosemary up very finely.
2. Store in a glass jar.

47: Rosemary Lavender Body Scrub

Ingredients:

- 2 cups Epsom salt
- 1 cup organic extra-virgin coconut oil
- 10-15 drops Lavender essential oil
- Sprig of fresh rosemary (optional)

Directions:

1. Combine all ingredients.
2. Use and store leftovers in a– you guessed it– glass jar!

48: Rosemary Sage Body Scrub

Ingredients:

- 1 cup sweet almond oil
- 2 cups sea salt
- rosemary essential oil
- sage essential oil

Directions:

1. Put the salt into the jar.
2. Slowly add the sweet almond (you might need less, just add enough so it's wet but not runny!).
3. Add six drops of your essential oils.
4. Store and use!

49: Garlic & Oatmeal Scrub for Blackheads & Whiteheads

Ingredients:

- 2 cloves of crushed garlic
- 1 tablespoon of ground oatmeal
- 1 drop of Tea Tree essential oil
- 2-3 drops of lemon juice
- Honey

Directions:

1. Mix everything together, adding only enough honey to get a paste-like consistency.
2. Apply to areas of your face effected with blackheads and whiteheads!

50: Thyme & Sage Scrub

Ingredients:

- 1 cup sea salt
- 1 tablespoon dried, ground thyme
- 1 tablespoon dried, ground sage
- ¼ cup oil (olive, grapeseed, jojoba)
- ½ lemon, juiced
- 1 tablespoon honey

Directions:

1. Blend all of the ingredients.
2. Scrub on, and rinse off!

Thank You!

Thank you so much for purchasing this book, I do hope you enjoyed it! If you love clean, natural recipes, go to my blog for more… EmmasTake.WordPress.com. I love sharing recipes and beauty advice there, so be sure to check it out.

Thank you again for purchasing, if you liked this book, please tell your friends and family and take a moment to leave a review! It would mean the world to me ☺

Wishing you a happy time,

Emma

Want more?

Go to EmmasTake.WordPress.com for beauty, health, and lifestyle advice from Emma. Also make sure to check out some of Emma's other books...

- 50 Best Body Butter Recipes
- 50 Best Vegetarian Recipes
- 50 Best Vegan Recipes
- 50 Best Raw Vegan Recipes
- 50 Best Paleo Recipes
- 50 Best Breakfast Dish Recipes
- 50 Best Microwave Dessert Recipes
- 50 Best Chocolate Dessert Recipes
- 50 Best Gift Ideas Under $10
- 50 Best Gift Ideas under $25
- 50 Best Simple Sewing Projects